I0437070

Psoriasis Simple Treatment

By

GUSTAVO SANCHEZ

Copy right © 2012

Contents

For everyone that has struggle with this skin condition and had no success treating it.

Hi my name is Gustavo and I have psoriasis.

I have struggle with this condition for over 20 years. Thru many visits to dermatologist and naturalist plus doing my own personal research I have develop a way to control psoriasis.

You are probably saying how is it possible to come out with your own way to treat psoriasis? Like I said before, thru many visits to dermatologist, naturalist, book research and articles found online I was able to come out with a simple plan to decrease breakouts, soothe skin and believe me it works, just keep reading.

Here is the first thing I did whenever anyone finds something wrong with their skin, run to a dermatologist.

Now I am not saying a dermatologist is not a good source to find answers about skin conditions but they are not the only source to get answers either.

I found out that dermatologist know the scientific side of how to determine what type of skin condition an individual is suffering from and the kind of medicine, cream or ointment to use for treatment, that's why no matter how many different dermatologist I visited I kept ending up with creams or ointments that would not work properly and this was becoming frustrating.

By the way I did found an ointment that really works after many years of trying different kinds, I will give you details about it later on.

Second thing I tried after getting nowhere with a dermatologist was to try a naturalist, now here I was getting closer to my answer in solving the psoriasis problem.

The difference with a naturalist is that they find out what is causing the skin condition by first doing a cleanse and providing you with a very strict diet that to me was impossible to stick with, I had to cut seasonings, meats, a whole bunch of food just to be left with plain vegies and tasteless soups that made me drop so much pounds even my friends were worry about my health.

Although I did not commit to any naturalist diet, I did how ever found out from them that some foods trigger psoriasis breakouts, I will tell you later about those foods.

Lastly after giving up any hope in finding any good treatment for my skin condition I decided to do some intense research, I read books on the subject and also found lots of internet articles that really helped me get a better understanding why certain things did work and others didn't. Finally I was in the right track to deal with psoriasis.

On the next page I will tell you what I learn from my experiences to come out with the treatment.

#1

My Dermatology answer

The cream or ointment that really work is called **TRIAMCINOLONE ACETONIDE OINTMENT USP, 0.1%** the brand name I use is **FOUGERA** but any other brand is good just make sure is the same ointment name.

From all the ointments I used this one is the only one that was able to heal my skin fast, I would apply a small amount to the affected skin area and the next day it was gone, is so good that it even works great on acne.

I recommend to apply small amounts of this ointment where you need it because is so oily that a small amount will cover a lot of skin area, do not go out on the sun or smoke cigars wen wearing this ointment, you might get burn.

For this ointment you will need a prescription from your dermatologist and regular price for 80 grams is around $20 or less, not bad for what it does.

One more thing, you need to use a mild shampoo and soap, I use shampoo 809 ESTRELLA and bar soap DALAN but any mild product will do.

#2

My Naturalist answer

Foods that need to be reduced in consumption are...

Milk, Coffee, Citric fruits and vegetables like **Oranges, Lemons, Tomatoes** are main ones**, Liquor, Fry food** and the top main KILLER **SUGAR** or **CORN SYRUP!!**

These foods are the cause of the break outs and intense itching that occurs when one of them is taken, some have stronger reaction to the skin than others and sugar is the most dangerous one in creating psoriasis break outs.

You can start by cutting down each of these little by little but if you are suffering from a severe skin itching and breaking I suggest to cut them in one shot, trust me you will see results almost instantly.

In time all the above foods can be consume again moderately, making sure not to overdo it to the point of breaking out but be very careful with **SUGAR** or **CORN SYRUP!!**

I found out every time Milk, Coffee, Citric fruits or vegies, fry food and even liquor was introduced in my body once in a while it had a minor effect on the skin but not **SUGAR!**

The minute **SUGAR** got in my body it completely had an instant reaction, triggering psoriasis in a matter of 24hrs or even faster, it did not matter what type of **SUGAR** product I consumed, sport drinks, bottle juices, table sugar, cookies, cake, corn syrup, all of them were making my skin itch and break!

If you need sweets in your diet then eat fresh fruits or fresh fruit juice, if that does not work then sweeten your drink with one tea spoon of sugar but nothing more than one and keep track of how this effects your skin!

#3

My Research
answer

After all the above was being done I found out that there was a need for extra prolong skin healing and that's when it was found that my body needed antioxidants and some sort of natural oil to intake so my skin can produce natural skin oil to fight the effects of dry skin done by Psoriasis, the answer? **FLAXSEED OIL**! Now you might say how bout **FISH OIL**? Yes you can use fish oil but **FLAXSEED** has the highest Omegas you can find and that's the main reason is so effective, now you might ask, what kind of flaxseed to buy? The answer is liquid soft gels, do not get the powder, you need the concentrated oil to work fast in your system and any brand will do, do not go by the most expensive brand because all you are paying for is the name brand, I usually get the Rite Aid or CVS brand because they are cheaper and bring a lot of soft gels.

By the way, before finding out about Flaxseed I was using YELLOW DOCK ROOT but stop using it after noticing that Flax was the only thing needed!

Almost forgot! Drink lots of water, this liquid cleans your body completely and try to drink water after every meal to help break down food in your intestines.

My conclusion

#1

Get the **TRIAMCINOLONE OINTMENT** and apply on affected area.

#2

Cut or consume less of **Milk**, **Coffee**, **Liquor**, **Citric** fruits or vegies like **Orange**, **Lemon**, **Tomatoes**, **Fry food** and do your best to stay away from **SUGAR** or **CORN SYRUP!!**

#3

Buy **FLAXSEED OIL** and take one soft gel daily.

#4

Drink lots of water after every meal or any time you feel thirsty, keep in mind the human body is 60% water so taking this liquid constantly keeps your entire system fresh!

In all I suggest to moderately start cutting down consumption of the things mention before but again if you need to get rid of that painful annoying skin condition fast just cut it all at once and start applying the ointment and drinking the Flaxseed, after your skin gets better you can start introducing the foods you like but be careful not to overdo it or you will end up where you started!

One last thing, results will vary from person to person but if follow thru step by step you will see how your skin will start to look better day by day.

Thank you for reading this manual and hope the best on your Psoriasis Simple Treatment.

www.ingramcontent.com/pod-product-compliance
Lightning Source LLC
Chambersburg PA
CBHW030105300526
45785CB00019B/2777